Healthy Eating made easy

A beginner's guide to Nutritious meals

JUSTINAH ADESEMOYE

ISBN: 9798396233584

DEDICATION

I dedicate this book to those who are eager to break free from old patterns and embrace the power of nutritious meals. May you discover inspiration, helpful hints, and delectable recipes on these pages, allowing you to make educated decisions and live a better lifestyle.

To my family and friends, Thank you for your constant encouragement and conviction in my passion for promoting well-being. Your love and encouragement have motivated my determination to share the information and insights contained inside these pages.

Thank you

CONTENTS

INTRODUCTION

I'm happy to welcome you to "Healthy Eating Made Easy: A Beginner's Guide to Nutritious Meals." Finding a way toward a healthy and balanced diet can be difficult in a society where we are continually inundated with fast food alternatives, processed snacks, and conflicting dietary recommendations. With the aid of a thorough manual provided in this book, you may embrace healthy eating with confidence and simplicity.

Firstly, We are all aware of the direct connection between what we eat and our physical and mental health. Our bodies are fueled by a nutrient-rich food, which also improves our energy levels and promotes overall health. In this book, we'll examine the value of a good diet and how it may improve all aspects of your life, from your disposition to your longevity.

Also, Starting a journey toward a healthy diet can be difficult at times. Perhaps you've run across challenges like having little time to prepare meals, reading product labels incorrectly, or believing that flavor must be sacrificed when eating healthfully. Be certain that we will address these frequent issues and dispel myths, giving you useful advice and empowering you to get past any obstacles in the way of living a better lifestyle.

The goal of "Healthy Eating Made Easy" is to become your go-to guide for establishing a solid foundation of wholesome eating practices. We will cover the fundamentals of nutrition throughout the chapters, assist you in creating a balanced plate, show you how to read food labels and ingredient lists, and provide helpful advice for savvy grocery shopping. We'll also go into batch cooking, meal planning, and healthy cooking techniques to give you the skills and knowledge you need to make smart decisions with ease.

We also recognize the value of convenience, so we've included quick and wholesome breakfast suggestions, healthy lunch and dinner recipes, and even snacks and desserts for those times when you want a treat but don't want to give up your objectives. This book's emphasis on developing long-term healthy eating habits rather than just quick fixes will help you maintain your success and continue to make wise decisions even after you graduate from the novice level.

By the time you finish reading this book, you'll have learned everything there is to know about nutrition, perfected the art of preparing balanced meals, and uncovered a ton of useful tips for leading a healthy lifestyle. On your path to a happier, healthier you, our goal is to inspire and assist you.

So let's set off on this thrilling journey together and learn how "Healthy Eating Made Easy" may change your life, one scrumptious and healthy meal at a time.

UNDERSTANDING THE BASICS OF NUTRITION

Understanding the fundamental components of nutrition is essential if you want to start a road toward good eating. The fundamentals of nutrition will be covered in detail in this chapter, along with information on fiber, water, and the importance of macronutrients, micronutrients, and other dietary components.

Macronutrients: Carbohydrates, Proteins, and Fats

Carbohydrates: Our bodies need carbohydrates as their main source of energy. We will examine the various kinds of carbohydrates, including simple and complex carbs, which can be found in refined sugars and entire grains, fruits, and vegetables. Learn how to choose wisely and include the proper amount of carbohydrates in each of your regular meals.

Proteins: Proteins are essential for tissue growth and repair, immune system support, and the regulation of many biological processes. Learn how to meet your protein needs by incorporating lean sources of protein into your diet, such as poultry, fish, lentils, and tofu.

Fats: There are various types of fats. Discover the various kinds of fats, including the good fat : monounsaturated and polyunsaturated found in foods like avocados, almonds, and fatty fish as well as the unhealthy fats : saturated and trans found in processed and fried meals. Learn how to make decisions that will promote your overall health and wellbeing.

Micronutrients: Vitamins and Minerals

Vitamins: Explore the B-vitamins, vitamin A, vitamin C, and other key vitamins that are needed for optimum health. Recognize their roles, the foods that contain them, and the significance of ensuring a balanced intake of these micronutrients.

Minerals: Find out how essential biological activities are supported by minerals like calcium, iron, magnesium, and potassium. Learn about foods that are high in certain minerals and how they help to keep the body healthy.

The Role of Fiber and Water in a Healthy Diet

Fiber: Recognize the role that dietary fiber plays in supporting appropriate weight control, enhancing digestive health, and preserving normal cholesterol levels. Learn about foods that are high in fiber, such as whole grains, legumes, fruits, and vegetables, and how to include them in your diet.

Water: Water is necessary for hydration, healthy digestion, absorption of nutrients, and general wellbeing.

Discover the value of remaining hydrated, how much water you ought to drink each day, and methods for increasing your water intake.

Gaining a thorough understanding of macronutrients, micronutrients, fiber, and water will provide you the information you need to make wise decisions while organizing and preparing your meals. Remember that a balanced diet contains each of these vital elements, giving your body the resources it requires to thrive.

To provide you with the knowledge necessary to prepare wholesome and filling meals, we will discuss practical methods for creating a balanced plate in the following chapter. Let's proceed with our journey toward healthy eating and learn how to balance our plates while also fueling our bodies for maximum wellbeing.

BUILDING A BALANCED PLATE

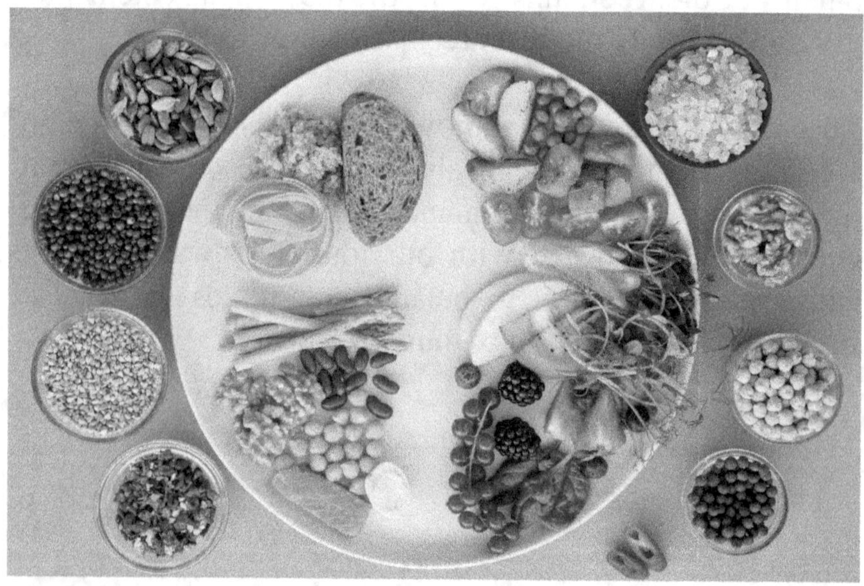

Understanding the idea of creating a balanced plate is crucial for achieving a healthy and nourishing diet. You will be led through the concepts of portion control, mindful eating, and the significance of including a range of food categories in your meals in this chapter. Your body will obtain the nutrients it needs for optimum health and well-being if you prepare balanced meals with the right quantities.

The Concept of Portion Control and Mindful Eating

Portion Control: Learn the value of portion control in preserving a healthy weight and avoiding overeating. Discover practical methods for determining the right serving sizes for various food groups, and practice identifying satiety cues to help you feel full without overeating.

Mindful Eating: Investigate the art of mindful eating, which is being totally present and conscious when eating. Discover ways to slow down, appreciate each meal, and develop a stronger relationship with your food. You may improve your whole dining experience and establish a healthier relationship with food by practicing mindful eating.

Understanding the Food Groups and Their Nutritional Benefits

Grains: Learn about the value of whole grains and their high fiber content. Learn how to include a range of whole grains in your meals, such as quinoa, brown rice, and whole-wheat bread.

Fruits and vegetables: Learn about the nutritional advantages of fruits and vegetables, which are brimming with vitamins, minerals, and fiber. To create a varied and vivid dish, consider several types, colors, and seasonal possibilities.

Proteins: Recognize the significance of including lean sources of protein in your meals, such as poultry, fish, lentils, and tofu. Learn the advantages of plant-based proteins and how to balance your protein intake for the best possible health.

Dairy or Dairy Alternatives: Examine how dairy products and dairy substitutes contribute to our intake of calcium, vitamin D, and other necessary nutrients. For your dietary preferences, find out about lactose-free and plant-based alternatives.

Fats and Oils: Recognize the function of healthy fats in your diet and develop the ability to distinguish between sources of healthy and bad fat. Learn the advantages of adding foods like avocados, almonds, seeds, and olive oil to your diet.

Making a Balanced Meal with the Right Portion

The Plate Method: Discover the useful and successful Plate Method, which involves splitting your plate into parts for several dietary groups. To make a plate that is both balanced and aesthetically pleasing, learn how to distribute the right amounts of veggies, proteins, whole grains, and fats.

Meal Planning Tips: Discover how to blend various food groups to make delicious and nutritionally sound recipes. For time savings and healthier options throughout the week, consider methods for incorporating leftovers and meal preparation.

Understanding the significance of balancing flavors and textures in your meals will help you make them more enjoyable. Learn how to utilize herbs, spices, and healthful sauces or dressings to improve flavor and provide variety.

You can prepare wholesome, well-balanced meals by being aware of portion control, engaging in mindful eating, and using a variety of food categories in the right amounts. In the following chapter, we'll delve into the subject of interpreting food labels and ingredient lists so that you can purchase with confidence. Let's continue on our path to a healthy diet so that we may learn how to interpret nutrition labels and choose the items that will be most beneficial to our wellbeing.

NAVIGATING FOOD LABELS AND INGREDIENTS

Making informed and healthy eating choices in today's food environment requires comprehending ingredient lists and analyzing food labels. This chapter will provide you the information and abilities to read food labels properly, spot hidden sugars, bad fats, and additives, and empower you to choose your groceries wisely.

How to Read and Interpret Nutrition Labels Effectively

Serving Sizes: Recognize the significance of serving sizes given on nutrition labels and discover how to calculate the ideal serving size for a specific meal.

Calories and Macronutrients: Learn how to read nutrition labels to determine whether the calorie count and information about the macronutrients (carbohydrates, proteins, and fats) correspond to your dietary objectives.

% Daily Value (%DV): Learn about the%DV and how it can be used to compare the nutritional value of different foods to your daily requirements.

Key Nutrients: Learn about the vital nutrients, including salt, fiber, vitamins, and minerals, as well as how to read the nutrition label to make sure you are getting the right amount of each.

Identifying Hidden Sugars, Unhealthy Fats, and Additives

Hidden Sugars: Learn how to spot added sugars on ingredient lists by being familiar with the numerous names they go by. Learn about the negative effects of excessive sugar consumption and how to minimize your intake.

Unhealthy Fats: Learn about the various harmful fats, including saturated and trans fats, and their detrimental effects on health. Choose foods with less unhealthy fats by becoming familiar with how to identify these fats on nutrition labels.

Additives and Preservatives: Learn how to recognize them on ingredient lists, as well as the common additives and preservatives found in food, and their potential health effects. Choose foods that have few additives or go for natural and minimally processed alternatives.

Making Informed Choices by Understanding Ingredient Lists

Ingredient Order: The order of the ingredients is based on their quantity. Learn to pay attention to the first few ingredients in a product because they are more prevalent.

Whole Foods and Natural Ingredients: Learn the advantages of choosing whole foods and natural ingredients, as well as how to spot them on ingredient lists. Recognize the benefits of selecting foods with recognizable and healthy ingredients.

Allergens and Sensitivities: Develop the ability to quickly scan ingredient lists for allergies or compounds that can cause reactions. Learn about common allergens and the need of being watchful when it comes to food safety.

You'll be able to shop with confidence if you learn how to decipher nutrition labels, spot hidden sugars, harmful fats, and additives, and comprehend ingredient lists. The issue of wise grocery shopping will be covered in the following chapter, and we'll provide you useful advice on how to organize and make a healthy grocery list. Let's continue our journey toward healthy eating, where we will equip you to choose wholesome options and pick the ideal ingredients for your well-being.

SMART GROCERY SHOPPING

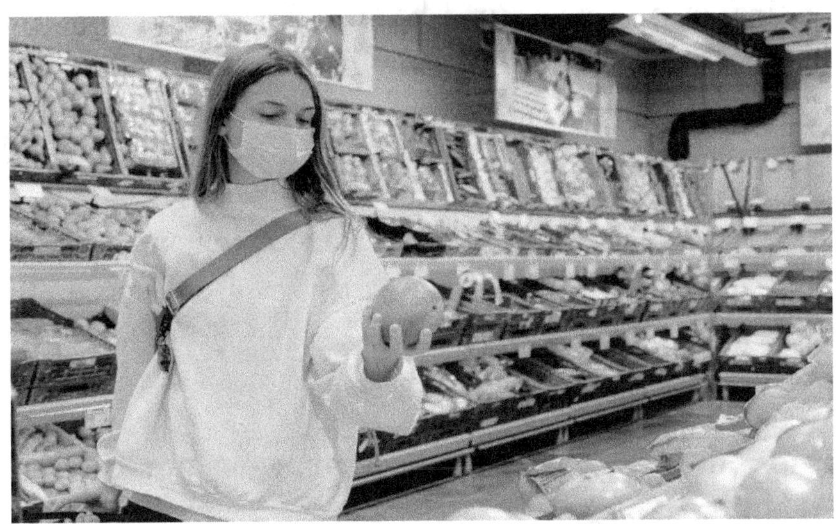

A vital component of keeping a balanced diet is smart food shopping. This chapter will walk you through the process of organizing and developing a nutritious grocery list, offer advice on how to buy smartly on a budget without sacrificing nutrition, and offer tactics for navigating the grocery store.

Planning and Creating a Healthy Grocery List

Assessing Your Needs: Look through your pantry, refrigerator, and freezer to see what needs to be restocked. Consider your weekly food plans and list the ingredients necessary to prepare wholesome meals.

By including a variety of fruits, vegetables, whole grains, lean proteins, and healthy fats, you can increase the nutritional value of your diet. To keep your meals varied and interesting, prioritize seasonal food and try out new components.

Plan your meals for the upcoming week so that you are aware of all the ingredients you will need. You may minimize impulsive purchases and lessen food waste by doing this.

Tips for Shopping in a Supermarket and Choosing Healthier Foods

Stick to the Perimeter: In a typical supermarket, the fresh vegetables, meats, dairy, and other whole foods are located around the perimeter. To include nutrient-dense ingredients in your meals, concentrate your buying mostly on these categories.

Read the Labels Cautiously: Use what you learned in Chapter 4 to effectively read and understand nutrition labels. Choose items with the fewest unhealthy fats, sugars, and additives possible. Choose whole food components over highly processed ones.

Choose Fresh and healthy Foods: Give fresh produce, lean meat, healthy grains, and minimally processed foods top priority. These options are typically more nutrient-dense and less likely to have extra sweets, bad fats, or artificial additives.

Shopping on a Budget Without Compromising Nutrition

Plan Ahead: Establish a spending limit for your grocery trips and schedule your meals appropriately. This will enable you to stay on track with your financial objectives and help you avoid impulsive purchases.

Buy Staples in quantity: Take into account buying grains, legumes, and frozen fruits and vegetables in quantity. Purchasing in bulk can save you money and give you products that can be used for several meals.

Compare Prices and Look for Sales: Spend some time looking for sales or discounts as well as comparing prices of comparable products. Think about buying store brands because they frequently provide comparable quality at a lesser price.

Always remember that healthy eating habits are built on sensible food shopping. You may make substantial progress towards attaining your health and wellness objectives by organizing and establishing a healthy food list, making wise decisions at the store, and shopping on a budget without sacrificing nutrition.

The issue of healthy cooking procedures will be covered in more detail in the following chapter, giving you useful information about methods that maintain nutrients and enhance flavors. Let's continue our path toward healthy eating so that we can discover how to cook scrumptious, filling meals while keeping our health in mind.

HEALTHY COOKING METHODS

The right cooking techniques are essential for keeping nutrients in tact and bringing out the best flavors in your food. This chapter will introduce you to a variety of nutrition-focused cooking methods, offer healthier substitutes for deep-frying and frying, and show you how to enhance flavors with herbs, spices, and nutritious marinades.

Introduction to Various Cooking Techniques that Preserve Nutrients

Steaming: a gentle cooking technique that preserves the vitamins, minerals, and vibrant colors of vegetables. Learn how to perfectly steam veggies while preserving their nutritious worth.

Sautéing and stir-frying: a rapid cooking with little oil. Learn how to cook food quickly, add veggies, proteins, and spices, and keep the nutrients in your food.

Understand how roasting and baking may result in scrumptious and wholesome foods. Learn how to bake lean proteins, roast veggies, and use dry heat to bring out tastes while preserving nutritional value.

Choosing Healthier Alternatives to Frying and Deep-Frying

Learn the pleasures of grilling, a technique that gives meats, vegetables, and even fruits smokey tastes. Learn how to marinate, season, and grill veggies and lean proteins to make recipes that are both tasty and healthy.

Oven-Baking: Acquire the skills to bake rather than fried food in your oven. Learn how to make baked alternatives to often fried items, such as breaded vegetables, oven-baked fries, and chicken tenders.

Investigate the idea of air frying as a healthier option to deep fried. Learn the advantages of air fryers, how they operate, and how to cook tasty foods that are crispy and low in oil.

Maximizing Flavors with Herbs, Spices, and Healthy Marinades

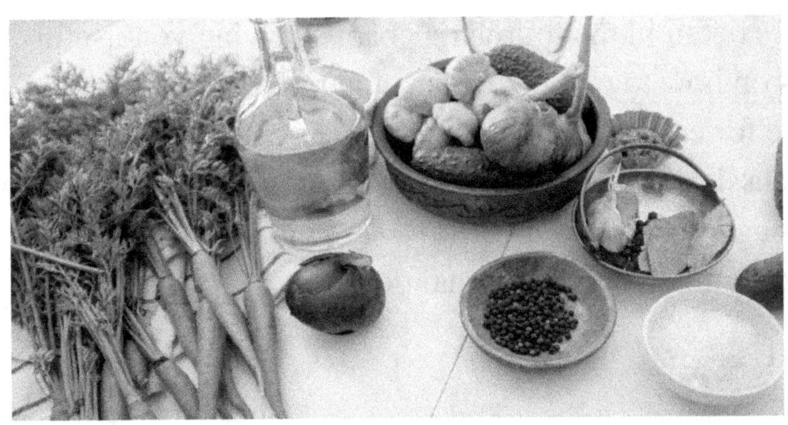

Discover the wide world of herbs and spices and how they may enhance your meals in "Herbs and Spices." Discover the therapeutic properties of various herbs and spices, and play around with flavor combinations to enhance the flavor of your food.

Healthy Marinades: Discover the technique of marinating to accentuate flavors and soften proteins. Learn how to make nutritious marinades using yogurt, citrus juices, herbs, spices, and natural sweeteners. To make tasty and wholesome meals, learn how to marinate meats, tofu, and veggies.

You may prepare delectable and nutrient-dense meals that promote your health by using cooking methods that preserve nutrients, selecting healthier alternatives to frying and deep-frying, and optimizing taste with herbs, spices, and healthy marinades.

We will discuss meal preparation and batch cooking in more detail in the following chapter, giving you useful tips on how to organize, plan, and make meals ahead of time for ease and effectiveness. Let's continue our discussion on healthy eating so that you can learn how to manage your time and effort in the kitchen while maintaining your nutritional goals.

MEAL PREPPING AND BATCH COOKING

Batch cooking and meal planning are effective techniques that can completely change the way you approach healthy eating. This chapter will cover how to plan and organize weekly meal preps, the advantages of meal preparation for time savings and staying on schedule, and advice on how to store, reheat, and preserve food freshness.

Benefits of Meal Prepping for Saving Time and Staying on Track

Time Savings: By setting aside a specified time each week to prepare meals in advance, you can learn how meal planning can help you save time throughout the week. Learn to simplify your cooking routine so you can take advantage of the ease of ready-to-eat prepared meals.

Explore how meal planning enables you to manage portion sizes and make deliberate choices regarding the contents and nutritional value of your meals in this section on portion management and healthy choices. You may minimize the probability of turning to unhealthy options by planning your meals in advance and making sure they are conveniently available.

Consistency and Accountability: Accept meal planning as a tool for maintaining your commitment to a balanced diet. By having pre-made meals on hand, you are less likely to give in to fast food or impulsive eating, encouraging a regular and conscientious approach to your nutrition.

Planning and Organizing Weekly Meal Preps

Menu Planning: Learn how to organize your meals for the week by taking your schedule, food choices, and nutritional requirements into account. Learn how to design balanced menus that include a range of food groups and flavors.

Batch Cooking: Study the idea of batch cooking, which entails making a variety of foods in large quantities to be eaten over the course of the week. To ensure you have adaptable ingredients that can be blended in many ways, gain knowledge into batch cooking processes for meats, cereals, and vegetables.

Efficient Kitchen Workflow: Acquire techniques for increasing your efficiency when preparing meals in the kitchen. To cut down on time and effort, learn proper kitchen tool use, ingredient organization, and cooking process optimization.

Tips for Storing, Reheating, and Maintaining Food Freshness

Proper Storage Containers: Recognize the significance of storing your food in appropriate containers to preserve its quality and freshness. Consider many possibilities, such as glass containers, containers with sections for meal preparation, and freezer-safe containers.

Labeling and Dating: To maintain correct rotation and prevent food waste, understand the value of labeling and dating your prepared meals. Learn how to properly label containers with information like as meal names, dates, and any ingredients or reheating instructions.

Reheating Methods: Learn the best methods for reheating prepared meals while preserving their flavor and texture. Learn which warming techniques are most effective for certain sorts of dishes by investigating several options such the stovetop, oven, microwave, and steam.

You can enjoy the time-saving advantages of having wholesome meals on hand by adopting meal planning and batch cooking. You may maintain your dietary objectives and take advantage of the convenience of tasty, nourishing meals throughout the week with careful planning and organization.

The importance of starting your day with a healthy meal

will be highlighted along with a range of quick and wholesome breakfast recipes and ideas in the following chapter, which will focus on quick and wholesome breakfast ideas. Let's continue our healthy eating adventure so that we can motivate you to start your mornings with energizing meals.

QUICK AND NUTRITIOUS BREAKFAST IDEAS

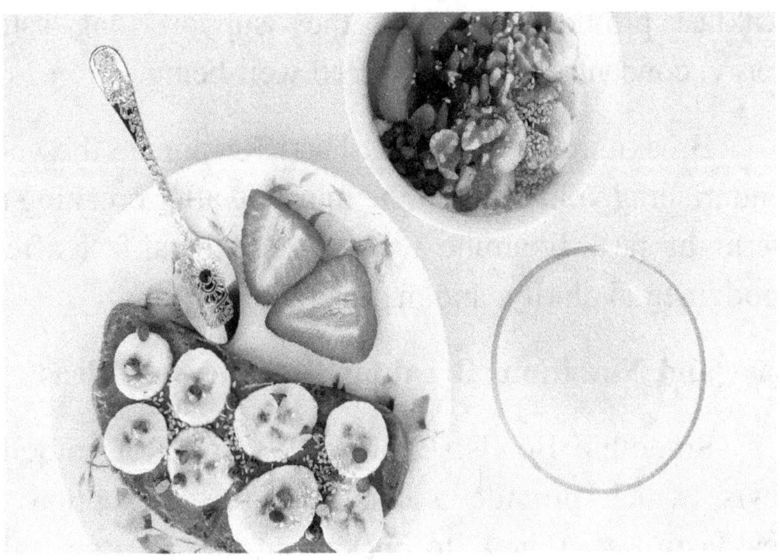

For good reason, breakfast is sometimes praised as the most significant meal of the day. We will discuss the significance of a healthy breakfast and how it affects energy levels in this chapter. We will also provide you a range of quick and wholesome breakfast dish ideas and suggestions, as well as advice on how to include protein, whole grains, and fruits and vegetables in your morning meal.

Importance of a Healthy Breakfast and Its Impact on Energy Levels

Fueling Your Body: Learn how a healthy breakfast creates the conditions for the best possible energy levels throughout the day. Learn about the vital nutrients a good breakfast provides and how they support long-lasting energy, concentration, and overall well-being.

Breaking the Overnight Fast: Recognize the value of nourishing your body in the morning after breaking the overnight fast. Examine how a good breakfast affects mood, mental clarity, and metabolism.

Easy and Nutritious Breakfast Recipes and Ideas

Smoothie Bowls: Explore the world of smoothie bowls, which provide a cool and flexible option for breakfast. Learn how to make nutrient-rich smoothie bases and how to add different fruits, nuts, seeds, and granola for texture and flavor.

Overnight Oats:Learn how to make overnight oats, a quick and easy breakfast option. For a delicious and filling bowl of oatmeal that is ready to eat in the morning, experiment with various flavor combinations and topping options.

Egg-Based Dishes:Learn how versatile eggs are and experiment with different ways to include them in your breakfast routine. Explore nutrient- and protein-rich options that can be tailored to your preferences, such as scrambled eggs with veggies, omelets, and egg muffins.

Tips for Incorporating Protein, Whole Grains, and Fruits/Vegetables

Breakfasts Rich in Protein: Investigate the significance of integrating protein into your morning meal and find out about various protein sources, for example, Greek yogurt, curds, nut spread, seeds, and lean meats. Find ideas for protein-rich breakfasts that support muscle growth and repair while also keeping you satisfied.

Whole Grains for Long-Term Power: Be aware of the advantages of including whole grains in your breakfast. Find out about choices, for example, entire grain bread, oats, quinoa, and entire grain cereals, and find imaginative ways of getting a charge out of them as a component of a nutritious morning dinner.

Vegetables and Fruits: Increase your nutrient intake by including fruits and vegetables in your breakfast. Investigate thoughts for integrating new or frozen natural products into smoothies, finishing off your short-term oats with berries, or adding vegetables to your egg-based dishes for added nutrients, minerals, and fiber.

You can start your day on the right foot, nourish your body, and set yourself up for success by recognizing the importance of a healthy breakfast, exploring easy and nutritious breakfast recipes, and incorporating protein, whole grains, and fruits and vegetables into your morning meal.

In the following part, we will dive into healthy lunch and supper recipes, giving you delightful and nutritious choices for balanced dinners. Let's continue our journey toward healthy eating by exploring dishes that nourish your body and taste buds while also being delicious and satisfying.

WHOLESOME LUNCH AND DINNER RECIPES

Enjoying scrumptious and substantial meals that promote your health and wellbeing is possible during lunch and supper. In this chapter, we'll look at savory and nutrient-dense lunch and dinner dishes, show you how to include lean meats, whole grains, and a variety of veggies in your meals, and give you advice on how to order takeaway or eat out more healthfully.

Flavorful and Nutritious Recipes for Well-Rounded Lunches and Dinners

Veggie-Loaded Buddha Bowl: Learn how to make a Buddha bowl that is colorful and rich in nutrients. Discover a wide range of colorful veggies, nutritious grains, and protein sources like tempeh, tofu, or grilled chicken, and discover how to balance flavors with dressings or sauces.

Mediterranean Quinoa Salad: Embrace the tastes of the Mediterranean by consuming a pleasant and refreshing quinoa salad. For a blast of flavor and nutrients, add vegetables like cherry tomatoes, cucumbers, olives, feta cheese, and a sprinkle of lemon vinaigrette.

Stir-Fried Noodles with Lean Protein: Discover the world of stir-fried noodles by combining healthy protein sources like shrimp, chicken, or tofu with a colorful array of veggies, whole grain noodles, or zucchini noodles to make a hearty and tasty dish.

Incorporating Lean Proteins, Whole Grains, and a Variety of Vegetables

Lean Protein Options: Recognize how crucial it is to include lean proteins in your lunch and evening meals. Learn how to prepare alternatives including skinless chicken breast, seafood, lentils, and plant-based protein sources while preserving their flavor and suppleness.

Whole Grain Goodness: Learn about the advantages of whole grains and how they contribute to fiber and sustained energy. For extra nutritious benefit, add whole grain ingredients like brown rice, quinoa, whole wheat pasta, or whole grain bread to your lunch and supper preparations.

Colorful Vegetable Variety: Accept the variety of veggies and try out various varieties, hues, and textures. To improve the nutritional value and aesthetic appeal of your meals, learn how to integrate leafy greens, cruciferous veggies, root vegetables, and colorful peppers.

Making Healthier Choices When Dining Out or Ordering Takeout

Menu Planning and Research: Learn how to make wise decisions whether eating out or ordering takeout. Learn how to study meals in advance, spot healthier selections, and make dietary goals-compatible changes or replacements.

Mindful Eating and Portion Control: Investigate methods for mindful eating whether eating out or getting takeaway. Learn to pay attention to your body's signals of hunger and fullness, enjoy every mouthful, and choose your portions carefully.

Smart Modifications: Learn how to improve the nutritional content of restaurant meals by making clever changes. Consider choices include asking for sauces or dressings on the side, selecting grilled or steamed foods, and switching out sides for healthier selections.

You can enjoy filling and nourishing lunches and dinners that support your overall well-being by looking into tasty and nutritious recipes, incorporating lean proteins, whole grains, and a variety of vegetables, and learning tips for choosing healthier options when dining out or ordering takeout.

In the following chapter, we'll dig into healthy sweets and snacks, giving you recipes for healthful desserts and scrumptious snacks that let you enjoy without straying from a well-balanced diet. Let's continue on our path to a healthy diet and learn how to enjoy delights in moderation while maintaining the nutritive and mouthwatering qualities of our snacks.

SNACKS AND DESSERTS FOR HEALTHY INDULGENCES

Snacks and sweets can be included in a balanced and nutritious diet. This chapter will cover mindful eating techniques for indulging in delights in moderation, healthy dessert recipes employing natural sweeteners and better-for-you ingredients, and smart snacking alternatives to quell cravings and increase energy.

Smart Snacking Options to Curb Cravings and Boost Energy

Nutrient-Dense Snack Ideas: Learn about several nutrient-dense foods that give you energy and sate your desires. Consider alternatives like Greek yogurt with berries, raw or roasted nuts and seeds, veggie sticks with hummus, or homemade energy snacks.

Balanced Snack Combinations: Learn how to combine a variety of macronutrients in balanced snack combinations, such as cottage cheese or hard-boiled eggs with whole-grain crackers or a little amount of almonds for a filling and nutritious snack.

Wholesome Dessert Recipes Using Natural Sweeteners and Healthier Ingredients

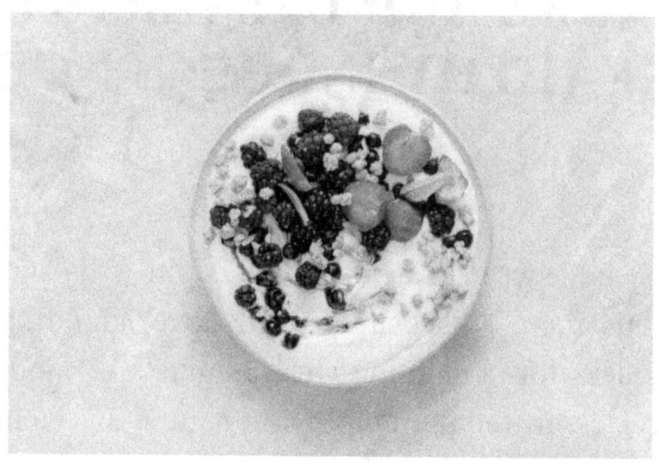

Fruit-based Desserts: Make delectable sweets like baked apples with cinnamon, fruit salads with a drizzle of honey or a squeeze of citrus, or homemade fruit popsicles using pureed fruits and yogurt by embracing the inherent sweetness of fruits.

Healthier Baking Alternatives: Consider whole grain flours like almond or oat flour and natural sweeteners like maple syrup, honey, or mashed bananas as healthier alternatives to processed flours and sugars while baking. Use these ingredients to create recipes for nutrient-dense cookies, energy balls, or muffins.

Mindful Eating Strategies for Enjoying Treats in Moderation

Portion Control and Mindful Indulgence: When it comes to savoring desserts and snacks, practice mindful eating. Practice portion management by enjoying smaller servings, paying attention to the flavor and texture of each mouthful, and letting yourself indulge guilt-free.

Conscious Treat Selection: Develop a deliberate approach to picking treats by selecting desserts or nibbles that actually make you happy and satisfied. Think on the quality of the foods, choose homemade dishes when you can, and pay attention to your body's hunger and fullness cues.

You may enjoy snacks and sweets while keeping a balanced approach to healthy eating by looking into smart snacking alternatives, including nourishing dessert recipes, and adopting mindful eating techniques.

The following chapter will cover long-term healthy eating patterns and provide you tips for continuing a diet that is healthy after the beginning stage. Let's continue on our path to a healthy, sustainable lifestyle, where we will look at how to overcome challenges, maintain motivation, and combine physical activity for overall wellness.

LONG-TERM HEALTHY EATING HABITS

Maintaining a healthy diet involves adopting long-term behaviors that promote your general wellbeing, not just making short-term adjustments. This chapter will include techniques for keeping up a healthy diet after the learning phase, cover ways to overcome setbacks and retain motivation, and place emphasis on the value of including exercise and physical activity for general heath.

Strategies for Maintaining a Healthy Diet Beyond the Beginner Stage

Consistency and Sustainability:Concentrate on developing a long-term dietary strategy that you can stick to. Focus on being consistent with your healthy food selections, meal planning, and adoption of a balanced strategy that fits your tastes and way of life.

Mindful Eating as a Lifestyle:Continue to cultivate the lifetime habit of mindful eating. During meals, pay attention to your body's signals of hunger and fullness, enjoy every bite, and remain in the present. By doing this, you may develop a healthy connection with food and enjoy meals more.

Overcoming Obstacles and Staying Motivated

Meal Planning and Preparation:Continue to plan and prepare your meals in advance to stay organized. This makes it easier for you to control your eating and guarantees that there are always wholesome food selections accessible. To keep your meals intriguing and pleasurable, try out different dishes and flavors.

Handling Social Situations: Make deliberate decisions when navigating social events and eating out. Be clear about your nutritional needs and preferences with those around you, put more emphasis on the people and the discussion than simply the food, and achieve balance by eating in moderation guilt-free.

Dealing with Setbacks: Recognize that setbacks do occur, and consider them opportunities for growth rather than failures. If you stray from your healthy eating plan, be kind to yourself and quickly get back on track. Keep in mind that growth is not always straight forward and that every day presents a fresh chance to make healthy decisions.

Incorporating Exercise and Physical Activity for Overall Wellness

Finding Activities You Enjoy: Engage in physical activities you actually like, whether it's yoga, cycling, swimming, dancing, or brisk walking. To make it simpler to integrate regular exercise into your schedule, find activities that suit your interests and lifestyle.

Setting Realistic Goals: Set attainable exercise objectives that suit your skills and interests. Start with manageable goals, then progressively boost the length or intensity of your exercises. To stay motivated, celebrate your accomplishments and monitor your development.

Creating an Active Lifestyle:Incorporate physical activity into your everyday life by looking for opportunities to do so. To make exercise a fun and sociable experience, use the stairs instead of the elevator, walk or bike to local locations, indulge in active hobbies, or join a group class or sports team.

You may establish long-term good eating habits and attain total wellbeing by putting techniques for keeping a balanced diet into practice, overcoming hurdles, and including exercise and physical activity into your daily routine.

In the last chapter, we'll wrap up our trip with a summary of the most important ideas discussed in the book, give inspiration and encouragement for you to keep working toward a healthy diet, and provide extra resources and references for future research. Let's conclude our discussion of healthy eating by recognizing your accomplishments and encouraging you to keep moving forward in your quest for a full and energized life.

CONCLUSION

Greetings and congratulations for finishing "Healthy Eating Made Easy: A Beginner's Guide to Nutritious Meals." We've looked at the fundamentals of healthy eating throughout this book and given you useful advice, recipes, and methods to help you start living a fed and active life. In this last chapter, we will summarize the most important ideas discussed, present more resources and references for further research, and motivate and inspire you to continue your journey.

Recap of Key Points Covered in the Book

Importance of Healthy Eating: We discussed how healthy eating contributes to overall well-being, boosts energy levels, supports a strong immune system, and reduces the risk of chronic diseases.

Basics of Nutrition: You learned about macronutrients (carbohydrates, proteins, and fats), micronutrients (vitamins and minerals), and the role of fiber and water in maintaining a healthy diet.

Building a Balanced Plate:We looked at the idea of portion management, categorizing foods, and putting together balanced meals with the right ratios.

Navigating Food Labels and Ingredients: You gained knowledge on how to read nutrition labels effectively, identify hidden sugars, unhealthy fats, and additives, and make informed choices by understanding ingredient lists.

Smart Grocery Shopping:We offered advice on creating a nutritious shopping list, utilizing the supermarket's layout to create healthier selections, and shopping on a budget without sacrificing nutrition.

Healthy Cooking Methods: You discovered various cooking techniques that preserve nutrients, learned about healthier alternatives to frying and deep-frying, and explored ways to maximize flavors with herbs, spices, and healthy marinades.

Meal Prepping and Batch Cooking: We highlighted the benefits of meal prepping for saving time and staying on track, discussed planning and organizing weekly meal preps, and provided tips for storing, reheating, and maintaining food freshness.

Quick and Nutritious Breakfast Ideas: You studied the significance of a healthy breakfast and its effect on energy levels, gained simple and nourishing breakfast dish ideas, and discovered how to include protein, whole grains, fruits, and vegetables in your morning meals.

Wholesome Lunch and Dinner Recipes: In addition to emphasizing the value of include lean meats, whole grains, and a range of veggies, we also presented tasty and nutrient-dense recipes for balanced lunches and dinners. We also gave advice on how to make better decisions while eating out or getting takeout.

Snacks and Desserts for Healthy Indulgences: You learned how to make healthful desserts with natural sweeteners and healthier ingredients, gained mindful eating techniques for indulging in delights in moderation, and learned smart snacking alternatives to squelch cravings and increase energy.

Long-Term Healthy Eating Habits: We covered methods for keeping up a healthy diet through the starter stage, provided advice for overcoming challenges and retaining motivation, and emphasized the need of include physical activity and exercise for general heath.

Encouragement and Inspiration for Readers' Journey Towards Healthier Eating

Taking the first step toward healthy eating is a transforming and personal experience. You must be patient and gentle to yourself along the journey because development takes time. Celebrate all of your accomplishments, no matter how large or small, and embrace the little wins. Focus on the good improvements you see, such as greater energy, a better mood, or better general health, to stay motivated. If you want to share experiences, swap ideas, and find inspiration, surround yourself with a supportive group of people, whether they are close friends, family, or internet forums.

Your dietary decisions give you the ability to transform your life for the better. Remember that eating healthily is about fueling your body with good, tasty meals rather than about limitation or deprivation. Enjoy the process of cooking, try out different tastes, and enjoy each bite. Keep in mind that your path to better eating is distinctive, and it's crucial to choose a strategy that fits your own tastes, requirements, and way of life.

We appreciate you coming along with us on this educational quest towards a healthy diet. Accept what you've learned, put it into practice, and take advantage of the amazing advantages of a healthy body and mind. May your journey be enriched with brilliant tastes, a surplus of energy, and a revitalized sense of wellbeing.

I hope you have a lifetime of delicious food and good health!

[Justinah Adesemoye]

ABOUT THE AUTHOR

Justinah Adesemoye, The author of "Healthy Eating Made Easy: A Beginner's Guide to Nutritious Meals," is a passionate advocate for healthy living and motivating people to make great changes in their life.

She has devoted years of research and personal experience to understanding the tremendous influence of good food on overall health and energy and has a great enthusiasm for nutrition and well-being.